The New War on Cancer

How mRNA Technology is Revolutionizing Treatment

Alexandra Everest

Copyright

Copyright © 2024 Alexandra Everest

All rights reserved. No part of this publication may be reproduced, distributed, or transmitted in any form or by any means, including photocopying, recording, or other electronic or mechanical methods, without the prior written permission of the publisher, except in the case of brief quotations embodied in critical reviews and certain other non-commercial uses permitted by copyright law.

Disclaimer: The information provided in this book is for educational and informational purposes only. It is not intended as a substitute for professional medical advice, diagnosis, or treatment. Always seek the advice of your physician or other qualified health provider with any questions you may have regarding a medical condition.

Table of Content

CHAPTER 1	**4**
THE MRNA REVOLUTION	**4**
The Science Behind mRNA: How It Works	4
The Role of mRNA in Combating COVID-19	8
Translating Success: From Virus to Cancer	11
CHAPTER 2	**14**
INSIDE THE CLINICAL TRIAL	**14**
Understanding Clinical Trials: Phases and Protocols	14
The BNT116 Vaccine: A Game-Changer for Lung Cancer?	17
CHAPTER 3	**20**
THE IMMUNE SYSTEM UNLEASHED	**20**
Immunotherapy: An Overview	20
How mRNA Vaccines Train the Immune System	24
Expert Opinions: The Potential of mRNA in Cancer Treatment	26
CHAPTER 4	**30**
CHALLENGES AND CONTROVERSIES	**30**
Balancing Hope and Hype: The Reality of mRNA Cancer Vaccines	30
Side Effects and Safety: What We Know So Far	33
Ethical Considerations in Experimental Treatments	35
CHAPTER 5	**39**
THE FUTURE OF CANCER TREATMENT	**39**
Scaling Up: From Trials to Standard Treatment	39
The Global Impact: What This Means for Cancer Patients Worldwide	42

Next Steps in mRNA Research   45
CONCLUSION   **50**

CHAPTER 1

THE MRNA REVOLUTION

The Science Behind mRNA: How It Works

The journey of messenger RNA, or mRNA, from a relatively obscure molecule to the forefront of medical innovation is nothing short of extraordinary. To understand its significance in cancer treatment, it's essential first to grasp the basics of how mRNA functions within the body.

Messenger RNA is a single-stranded molecule that carries genetic instructions from DNA to the cell's machinery for making proteins. In simpler terms, mRNA acts as a messenger, taking the information encoded in DNA—the blueprint of life—and delivering it to the cell's ribosomes, the molecular machines responsible for building proteins. These proteins are the workhorses of the cell, involved in virtually every function, from providing structural support to facilitating biochemical reactions.

For decades, scientists understood the fundamental role of mRNA in cellular biology, but the challenge was harnessing this molecule for therapeutic purposes. The idea of using mRNA as a medical tool, especially as a vaccine, faced significant hurdles. mRNA is inherently unstable and easily degraded by the body's natural defenses, which made it difficult to use as a reliable delivery system for therapeutic instructions.

However, through years of research and technological advancements, scientists developed methods to stabilize mRNA and deliver it effectively into cells. This breakthrough paved the way for the development of mRNA vaccines, which work by introducing a piece of mRNA into the body that encodes a protein unique to a particular virus or, in the case of cancer, a specific tumor. The cell's machinery reads the mRNA instructions and produces the protein, which is then recognized by the immune system as foreign. This triggers an immune response, effectively teaching the body to recognize and fight the virus or cancer cells in the future.

The beauty of mRNA technology lies in its adaptability and precision. Unlike traditional vaccines that rely on weakened or inactivated forms of viruses, mRNA vaccines are entirely synthetic and can be rapidly developed and adjusted. This allows for a more targeted approach to immunization, with the potential to customize treatments for individual patients based on their unique genetic makeup or the specific characteristics of their disease.

The concept of using mRNA to fight diseases like cancer is revolutionary. By delivering mRNA that encodes tumor-specific antigens—proteins found on the surface of cancer cells—scientists can essentially train the immune system to seek out and destroy cancer cells with remarkable precision. This approach not only offers a new line of defense against cancer but also minimizes the collateral damage to healthy cells, a common issue with conventional treatments like chemotherapy and radiation.

The Role of mRNA in Combating COVID-19

The COVID-19 pandemic thrust mRNA technology into the global spotlight, demonstrating its potential on a scale never before seen. Before the pandemic, mRNA vaccines were largely theoretical, with ongoing research but no widespread applications. However, the urgent need for a vaccine to combat the rapidly spreading SARS-CoV-2 virus accelerated the development and deployment of mRNA vaccines, marking a turning point in medical history.

BioNTech, a German biotechnology company, in collaboration with Pfizer, became one of the first to successfully develop and roll out an mRNA-based COVID-19 vaccine. The vaccine, known as BNT162b2, was revolutionary not only because it was the first mRNA vaccine to be approved for emergency use, but also because of how quickly it was developed. The traditional timeline for vaccine development spans several years, if not decades. Yet, the BNT162b2 vaccine was developed, tested, and brought to market in less than a year—a feat made possible by the flexibility and speed of mRNA technology.

The mechanism of the COVID-19 mRNA vaccine is straightforward: it contains mRNA that encodes the spike protein of the SARS-CoV-2 virus, the protein that allows the virus to enter human cells. Once injected, the mRNA instructs cells in the body to produce the spike protein, which is harmless on its own but prompts the immune system to generate a response. The immune system then "remembers" this spike protein, allowing it to mount a rapid and effective defense if exposed to the actual virus.

The success of mRNA vaccines in combating COVID-19 had profound implications for the future of vaccine development and infectious disease control. For the first time, scientists had a platform that could be rapidly adapted to emerging pathogens, offering hope in the face of future pandemics. But beyond infectious diseases, the success of these vaccines also rekindled interest in using mRNA technology to tackle other challenging diseases, including cancer.

Translating Success: From Virus to Cancer

The leap from using mRNA technology to combat infectious diseases to using it as a weapon against cancer represents one of the most exciting frontiers in modern medicine. The principles are similar: in both cases, the goal is to teach the immune system to recognize and destroy harmful cells. But cancer presents a unique set of challenges.

Unlike viruses, which are foreign invaders that the immune system is designed to attack, cancer cells are more insidious. They originate from the body's own cells, meaning the immune system often fails to recognize them as threats. This is one reason why cancer can be so difficult to treat—by the time the immune system realizes something is wrong, the cancer may have already spread.

The key to overcoming this challenge lies in identifying specific antigens—proteins or other molecules found on the surface of cancer cells but not on healthy cells. These antigens act as "flags" that can be used to direct the immune system to the right target. mRNA vaccines like BNT116 work by encoding these cancer-specific antigens, effectively turning the immune system into a precision-guided missile capable of seeking out and destroying cancer cells wherever they may be hiding.

Moreover, mRNA technology offers the potential for personalized medicine. In theory, an mRNA vaccine could be tailored to the specific genetic makeup of an individual's tumor, creating a bespoke treatment that is uniquely suited to their needs. This level of precision is unprecedented in cancer treatment and represents the future of oncology.

The journey from virus to cancer treatment is still in its early stages, but the success of mRNA vaccines against COVID-19 has provided a solid foundation for future developments. Clinical trials like the one Janusz participated in are crucial steps in this journey, as they help scientists gather the data needed to refine and improve these treatments.

CHAPTER 2

INSIDE THE CLINICAL TRIAL

Understanding Clinical Trials: Phases and Protocols

Clinical trials are the cornerstone of medical research, serving as the critical step between the development of new treatments and their approval for widespread use.

Clinical trials are typically divided into four phases, each with a specific goal and protocol.

Phase 1 trials, are the first step in testing a new treatment in humans. The primary focus of Phase 1 is to assess safety—determining the appropriate dosage, identifying potential side effects, and understanding how the treatment interacts with the human body. These trials are usually small, involving a limited number of participants who are closely monitored throughout the process.

The BNT116 vaccine was a novel treatment, and while it had shown promise in preclinical studies, its effects in humans were still largely unknown. The data gathered from participants would provide the foundation for future research, helping to determine whether the vaccine could move on to the next stages of development.

Phase 2 trials expand on the findings from Phase 1, focusing on the treatment's efficacy—whether it actually works in combating the disease it is designed to treat. These trials involve more participants and are designed to further assess safety while beginning to evaluate the treatment's effectiveness.

Phase 3 trials are even larger, often involving thousands of participants across multiple locations. These trials compare the new treatment to the current standard of care, gathering comprehensive data on its effectiveness, safety, and potential side effects. Successful Phase 3 trials are a prerequisite for regulatory approval.

Phase 4 trials occur after a treatment has been approved and brought to market. These trials continue to monitor the treatment's long-term effects, ensuring that it remains safe and effective in a broader population.

The BNT116 Vaccine: A Game-Changer for Lung Cancer?

The BNT116 vaccine, developed by BioNTech, represented a new frontier in cancer treatment. Utilizing the same mRNA technology that had proven so effective against COVID-19, this vaccine was specifically designed to target non-small cell lung cancer (NSCLC), the most common and deadly form of lung cancer.

The science behind BNT116 was both innovative and complex. At its core, the vaccine worked by delivering synthetic mRNA sequences into the body. These sequences encoded specific antigens—proteins found on the surface of NSCLC cells. Once inside the body, the mRNA instructed cells to produce these antigens, effectively turning the patient's own cells into factories that produced cancer-specific markers. The immune system, recognizing these markers as foreign, would then mount an attack against any cells displaying them, including the cancer cells.

This approach was revolutionary for several reasons. First, it offered a level of precision that traditional treatments like chemotherapy and radiation could not match. While these conventional treatments often kill both cancerous and healthy cells, leading to severe side effects, the BNT116 vaccine was designed to target only the cancer cells, leaving healthy tissue unharmed.

Second, the mRNA platform allowed for rapid development and customization. In theory, the vaccine could be tailored to the unique genetic profile of an individual's tumor, creating a personalized treatment that was far more effective than a one-size-fits-all approach. This adaptability was one of the reasons why mRNA technology was so promising, not just for cancer treatment but for a wide range of diseases.

CHAPTER 3

THE IMMUNE SYSTEM UNLEASHED

Immunotherapy: An Overview

The human immune system is one of the most powerful and sophisticated defense mechanisms known to science. It is a complex network of cells, tissues, and organs that work together to protect the body from harmful invaders such as viruses, bacteria, and other pathogens. However, the immune system's role extends beyond simply fighting off infections—it also plays a crucial part in identifying and eliminating abnormal cells, including those that can turn into cancer.

Immunotherapy is a form of treatment that leverages the body's immune system to fight diseases, including cancer. Unlike traditional treatments like chemotherapy and radiation, which target cancer cells directly but can also damage healthy cells, immunotherapy works by enhancing or restoring the immune system's ability to recognize and attack cancer cells.

There are several types of immunotherapy, each with a different mechanism of action:

1. **Checkpoint Inhibitors**: These drugs work by blocking the proteins that prevent the

immune system from attacking cancer cells. Cancer cells often exploit these proteins, known as checkpoints, to avoid detection. By inhibiting these checkpoints, the immune system can better recognize and destroy cancer cells.

2. **Adoptive Cell Therapy**: This approach involves collecting and using the patient's own immune cells, which are modified or enhanced in a laboratory to better fight cancer. The modified cells are then infused back into the patient, where they seek out and attack cancer cells.

3. **Cytokines**: These are signaling proteins that help boost the immune system's response to cancer. Cytokines can stimulate the growth of immune cells and increase their ability to attack cancer cells.

4. **Cancer Vaccines**: Unlike vaccines that prevent infections, cancer vaccines are designed to treat existing cancers. These vaccines work by training the immune system to recognize and attack cancer cells, often by introducing tumor-specific antigens that act as targets for immune cells.

Immunotherapy has revolutionized cancer treatment in recent years, offering new hope to patients with cancers that were once considered untreatable. However, not all patients respond to immunotherapy, and the reasons for this are still being studied. The success of immunotherapy depends on various factors, including the type of cancer, the patient's overall health, and the ability of the immune system to recognize the cancer cells as a threat.

How mRNA Vaccines Train the Immune System

The BNT116 vaccine represents a new frontier in immunotherapy. At the heart of this vaccine is messenger RNA (mRNA), a molecule that serves as a set of instructions for the immune system. Unlike traditional vaccines, which often use weakened or inactivated forms of a virus, mRNA vaccines work by providing the body with the genetic information needed to produce specific proteins—proteins that are found on the surface of cancer cells.

Here's how it works:

1. **Delivery of mRNA**: The vaccine is administered via injection, delivering the mRNA into the body's cells. Once inside, the mRNA instructs the cells to produce proteins that mimic the antigens found on the surface of cancer cells. These proteins

are harmless on their own, but they serve a critical purpose.

2. **Production of Antigens**: The cells begin to produce the antigens encoded by the mRNA. These antigens are then displayed on the cell's surface, where they can be recognized by the immune system.

3. **Immune System Activation**: The immune system, detecting these foreign antigens, responds by activating T-cells, a type of white blood cell that plays a key role in the immune response. The T-cells are trained to recognize and attack cells displaying these antigens, which in the context of the vaccine, are cancer cells.

4. **Memory Formation**: One of the most powerful aspects of the immune system is its ability to remember previous encounters with pathogens. After the initial immune

response, some T-cells become memory cells, which remain in the body long after the vaccine is administered. These memory cells enable the immune system to mount a faster and more robust response if it encounters the cancer cells again.

The BNT116 vaccine specifically targets non-small cell lung cancer (NSCLC), one of the most common and deadly forms of lung cancer. By introducing mRNA sequences that encode for antigens unique to NSCLC cells, the vaccine aims to train the immune system to seek out and destroy these cancer cells with precision.

Expert Opinions: The Potential of mRNA in Cancer Treatment

The success of mRNA vaccines in combating COVID-19 has sparked a wave of interest in their potential applications beyond infectious diseases. Leading experts in oncology and immunology are now exploring how this technology could be harnessed to revolutionize cancer treatment.

Dr. Siow Ming Lee, the clinical lead for the UK arm of the BNT116 trial, is one such expert. With decades of experience in lung cancer research, Dr. Lee has seen firsthand the limitations of traditional treatments. "When I started in the 1990s, nobody believed chemotherapy worked," he recalls. "We now know about 20-30% [of patients] stay alive with stage 4 with immunotherapy, and now we want to improve survival rates further. The potential of mRNA vaccines to provide that extra boost is incredibly exciting."

Dr. Lee's optimism is shared by Dr. Ugur Sahin and Dr. Özlem Türeci, the co-founders of BioNTech and pioneers of mRNA technology. In their view, the adaptability of mRNA vaccines is one of their greatest strengths. "The beauty of mRNA is that it's a platform technology," explains Dr. Sahin. "It can be quickly adapted to target different diseases by simply changing the mRNA sequence. This flexibility allows us to develop personalized treatments that are tailored to the specific genetic makeup of an individual's tumor."

This potential for personalization is particularly promising in the field of oncology, where no two tumors are exactly alike. Traditional treatments often take a one-size-fits-all approach, but mRNA technology opens the door to customized therapies that can be more effective and less harmful to healthy cells.

Dr. Michelle Mitchell, the chief executive of Cancer Research UK, also sees great promise in mRNA vaccines. "We're pleased to see that another cancer vaccine trial has opened in the UK, allowing more patients to access cutting-edge therapies," she says. "While this research is still in its early stages, the potential for mRNA vaccines to change the landscape of cancer treatment is undeniable."

Despite the excitement, experts are also cautious. The field of mRNA cancer vaccines is still in its infancy, and much remains to be learned about how to optimize these treatments for different types of cancer and different patient populations. Clinical trials like the one Janusz is participating in are critical for gathering the data needed to answer these questions and refine the technology.

CHAPTER 4

CHALLENGES AND CONTROVERSIES

Balancing Hope and Hype: The Reality of mRNA Cancer Vaccines

The development of mRNA cancer vaccines like BNT116 has sparked immense hope among patients, doctors, and researchers alike. The potential to train the body's immune system to target and destroy cancer cells with precision is revolutionary, offering a glimpse into a future where cancer might be managed or even cured without the debilitating side effects of traditional treatments. However, as with any new and emerging technology, it is crucial to balance optimism with a realistic understanding of the challenges that lie ahead.

One of the primary challenges in the field of mRNA cancer vaccines is the variability in how patients respond to treatment. While the concept of using mRNA to instruct the immune system to target cancer cells is scientifically sound, the human body is incredibly complex, and each patient's immune system is unique. What works well for one person may not be as effective for another. This variability makes it difficult to predict outcomes and complicates the process of developing a treatment that is universally effective.

Another significant challenge is the early stage of the research. Although the success of mRNA vaccines in the fight against COVID-19 has proven that this technology can be effective, cancer is a far more complicated target than a virus. Cancer cells are often adept at evading the immune system, and tumors can vary greatly not only between patients but also within the same patient over time. This heterogeneity makes it difficult to develop a one-size-fits-all vaccine, necessitating further research and the development of more sophisticated approaches.

The hype surrounding mRNA technology also presents a risk. In the aftermath of the COVID-19 pandemic, where mRNA vaccines played a critical role in controlling the virus, there is a tendency to view this technology as a panacea for all medical challenges.

However, it's important to recognize that while mRNA holds great promise, it is not without its limitations. The high expectations placed on this technology can lead to disappointment if it does not deliver immediate results in more complex applications like cancer treatment.

Side Effects and Safety: What We Know So Far

One of the most pressing concerns for any new treatment, particularly in the context of cancer, is its safety profile. Traditional cancer therapies like chemotherapy and radiation are notorious for their harsh side effects, which can include nausea, fatigue, hair loss, and an increased risk of infections due to weakened immunity. These side effects often add a significant burden to patients who are already dealing with the physical and emotional toll of cancer.

mRNA vaccines like BNT116 offer a potentially safer alternative by targeting cancer cells more precisely, thereby reducing damage to healthy cells. However, as with any new treatment, safety is not guaranteed, and potential side effects must be carefully studied and monitored.

During the early phases of clinical trials, close attention is paid to any adverse reactions experienced by patients. These can range from mild, such as injection site pain or mild flu-like symptoms, to more severe complications. The advantage of mRNA technology is its inherent design: because it uses synthetic instructions to produce antigens rather than introducing whole pathogens or live cells, it reduces the risk of unintended infections or immune reactions.

One of the critical aspects of the clinical trial process is the establishment of safety protocols. Participants are regularly monitored, with frequent check-ups and detailed records kept of any side effects or complications. This data is crucial not only for assessing the safety of the vaccine but also for refining the treatment and improving its efficacy.

The safety of mRNA cancer vaccines is a subject of intense scrutiny, both within the medical community and among the general public. While the potential benefits are immense, the risks must be carefully weighed, and transparent communication is key to maintaining public trust.

Ethical Considerations in Experimental Treatments

The use of experimental treatments in medicine, particularly in the context of life-threatening diseases like cancer, raises several ethical questions. These considerations are not only relevant to researchers and clinicians but also to patients who must make difficult decisions about their treatment options.

One of the primary ethical concerns is the balance between risk and benefit. Clinical trials, by their nature, involve a degree of uncertainty. For patients who are participating in a Phase 1 trial, the treatment is still in the early stages of development, and there is limited data on its effectiveness and safety. This raises the question of whether it is ethical to expose patients to potential risks when the benefits are not yet fully understood.

Informed consent is a critical component of addressing this ethical dilemma. However, the concept of informed consent is complex, especially when patients are in vulnerable positions, facing a disease with limited treatment options.

Another ethical issue is the equitable access to experimental treatments. Clinical trials are often conducted in specific locations, with limited spots available for participants. This can lead to disparities in who has access to potentially life-saving treatments. For instance, patients in rural areas or those without the means to travel to major research centers may be excluded from trials, raising concerns about fairness and equality in medical research.

Furthermore, there is the question of how to balance the needs of current patients with the broader goal of advancing medical knowledge. Clinical trials are essential for developing new treatments, but they also involve a degree of experimentation that may not always benefit the individual participant.

The ethical landscape of experimental treatments is further complicated by the involvement of pharmaceutical companies. These companies often fund and conduct clinical trials, and while their contributions are vital for advancing research, there is always a concern about conflicts of interest. Ensuring that trials are conducted transparently and with the primary focus on patient welfare is essential to maintaining ethical standards.

CHAPTER 5

THE FUTURE OF CANCER TREATMENT

Scaling Up: From Trials to Standard Treatment

The success of clinical trials raises an important question: how can these experimental treatments move from the controlled environment of a trial to becoming a standard part of cancer care?

The process of scaling up is complex and multifaceted, involving not only the refinement of the treatment itself but also the infrastructure and systems needed to deliver it on a large scale.

One of the first steps in this process is the completion of the clinical trial phases. For the BNT116 vaccine, the data collected from Phase 1 trials are crucial for understanding the vaccine's safety and preliminary efficacy. If these results are promising, the vaccine will move on to Phase 2 and Phase 3 trials, where it will be tested in larger populations and compared to existing treatments. Each phase is designed to gather more data, refine the treatment, and ensure that it is both safe and effective for a broad range of patients.

Once a treatment successfully passes through all phases of clinical trials, the next step is regulatory approval. In the UK, this involves rigorous evaluation by agencies such as the Medicines and Healthcare products Regulatory Agency (MHRA). The process is similar in other countries, with agencies like the U.S. Food and Drug Administration (FDA) or the European Medicines Agency (EMA) playing key roles. These regulatory bodies review the trial data, assess the risks and benefits of the treatment, and determine whether it can be approved for public use.

However, obtaining regulatory approval is just the beginning. To become a standard treatment, the vaccine must also be integrated into existing healthcare systems, which requires careful planning and coordination. This includes ensuring that healthcare providers are trained in administering the vaccine, that patients have access to the necessary facilities, and that the treatment is covered by insurance or national health services.

Moreover, the manufacturing and distribution of mRNA vaccines on a large scale present their own set of challenges. The production of mRNA vaccines requires specialized facilities that can produce the vaccine quickly and at high volumes. During the COVID-19 pandemic, companies like BioNTech and Moderna demonstrated that it was possible to rapidly scale up mRNA vaccine production, but doing so for cancer treatments, which may need to be tailored to individual patients, could be even more complex.

The Global Impact: What This Means for Cancer Patients Worldwide

The development of mRNA cancer vaccines has the potential to revolutionize cancer treatment on a global scale, offering new hope to patients who have limited options. However, the impact of this technology will depend on its accessibility and affordability, particularly in low- and middle-income countries where healthcare resources are often limited.

One of the most promising aspects of mRNA technology is its flexibility. Because mRNA vaccines can be rapidly designed and produced, they can be adapted to target different types of cancer and tailored to the genetic profiles of individual patients. This adaptability could make personalized cancer treatment a reality, allowing doctors to create vaccines that are specifically designed to target the unique characteristics of a patient's tumor.

However, the promise of personalized medicine also raises concerns about equity. While patients in high-income countries may have access to cutting-edge treatments, those in lower-income regions could be left behind if the infrastructure for producing and distributing mRNA vaccines is not established globally. This disparity could exacerbate existing inequalities in cancer care, where patients in poorer countries already face significant barriers to accessing treatment.

To address these challenges, international cooperation will be essential. Governments, pharmaceutical companies, and non-governmental organizations will need to work together to ensure that mRNA cancer vaccines are not only available but also affordable in all parts of the world. This could involve initiatives such as technology transfer agreements, where companies share their manufacturing processes with facilities in lower-income countries, or global health funds that subsidize the cost of vaccines for patients who cannot afford them.

The global impact of mRNA cancer vaccines also extends to how cancer is perceived and treated in different cultures. In many parts of the world, cancer is still seen as a death sentence, with limited treatment options and a heavy stigma attached to the disease. The introduction of new, effective treatments could change this narrative, offering hope and potentially reducing the fear and stigma associated with a cancer diagnosis

Next Steps in mRNA Research

While the focus of current mRNA research is largely on cancer and infectious diseases, the potential applications of this technology extend far beyond these areas. Scientists are exploring a wide range of possibilities, from treating autoimmune diseases to developing vaccines for other chronic conditions, such as diabetes or heart disease. The versatility of mRNA technology makes it a powerful tool in the search for new treatments and cures.

One of the next frontiers in mRNA research is the development of combination therapies that can target multiple aspects of a disease simultaneously. For example, researchers are investigating ways to combine mRNA vaccines with other forms of immunotherapy, such as checkpoint inhibitors, to enhance the overall effectiveness of treatment. These combination approaches could potentially overcome some of the limitations of single therapies, offering more comprehensive and durable responses in patients.

Another area of interest is the use of mRNA technology to treat genetic disorders. By delivering mRNA sequences that can correct or compensate for defective genes, scientists hope to develop treatments that address the root cause of these conditions rather than just managing the symptoms. This approach could have transformative effects on the treatment of diseases like cystic fibrosis, sickle cell anemia, and muscular dystrophy.

The continued advancement of mRNA technology will also require ongoing innovation in delivery methods. While the current vaccines are delivered via injection, researchers are exploring alternative delivery systems, such as nanoparticles, that could improve the efficiency and targeting of mRNA therapies. These advances could reduce the dosage required, minimize side effects, and allow for more precise delivery to specific tissues or organs.

The potential of mRNA research to expand beyond cancer treatment is both exciting and encouraging. It represents a broader vision of how medicine could evolve in the coming decades, with mRNA technology playing a central role in the development of new therapies across a wide range of diseases.

However, the future of mRNA research is not without challenges. One of the key issues is the need for sustained funding and support for basic research. While the success of mRNA vaccines during the COVID-19 pandemic has brought significant attention and investment to the field, it is crucial to maintain this momentum in the years to come. Continued investment in research and development is essential to unlocking the full potential of mRNA technology and ensuring that new treatments are brought to market.

CONCLUSION

The use of mRNA technology, which only a few years ago was largely experimental, has now emerged as a powerful tool in the fight against cancer. This technology's ability to train the immune system to recognize and destroy cancer cells with precision represents a new frontier in cancer treatment—one that holds the potential to transform the lives of millions of patients around the world.

But as we have seen, this journey is not without its challenges. The path from experimental treatment to standard care is long and complex, requiring rigorous testing, careful monitoring, and a deep commitment to patient safety. The uncertainties that accompany clinical trials, the variability in patient responses, and the ethical considerations of experimental treatments are all part of the broader landscape that must be navigated as we move forward.

Yet, despite these challenges, there is reason for optimism. The progress that has been made thus far is a powerful reminder of what can be achieved through dedication, collaboration, and a shared vision for a better future. The story of the BNT116 vaccine is not just a story of hope for those currently battling cancer—it is a story of hope for future generations, who may one day benefit from the advancements being made today.

Looking to the future, the possibilities for mRNA technology are vast. The success of the BNT116 vaccine in early trials offers a glimpse into a world where cancer treatment is more personalized, more effective, and less harmful. As research continues and new treatments are developed, we move closer to a time when cancer may no longer be the devastating diagnosis it is today. Instead, it may become a manageable condition—one that can be treated with the same precision and care that we now apply to other chronic diseases.

But this future will not come easily. It will require continued investment in research, ongoing support for clinical trials, and a commitment to ensuring that these advancements are accessible to all patients, regardless of where they live or their ability to pay. The fight against cancer is a global challenge, and it is one that demands a global response.

www.ingramcontent.com/pod-product-compliance
Lightning Source LLC
Chambersburg PA
CBHW070419230526
45471CB00006B/2877